CHRISTIAN CAREGIVING

PRACTICAL ADVICE FOR A HAPPY ENDING

BY

PATTI GREENE

Christian Caregiving: Practical Advice for a Happy Ending

Copyright @ 2018 by Patti Greene

Published by Awesome Librarian Press

Editor: Ellsworth Johnson

Photo Images: Photo 1-5, 7-8 Lightstock.com; Photo 6. Shutterstock.com

First Printing 2018

Printed in the United States of America

Scripture taken from the NEW AMERICAN STANDARD BIBLE, Revised Edition, © 1984, 1990, 2008 by AMG International, Inc. unless otherwise noted.
Trade Paperback
ISBN-13: 978-0692115381 (Awesome Librarian Press)
ISBN-10: 0692115382
Kindle Version ISBN-10: 0692115382

Library of Congress Cataloging-in-Publication Data
Name: Greene, Patti, author.
Title: Christian Caregiving: Practical Advice for a Happy Ending / Patti Greene.
Description: Awesome Librarian Press, 2018. Includes bibliographical references.
Subjects: LCSH: Caregiving. | Christian caregiving, a way of life. | Spiritual care. | Aging. | Home care.

This book is dedicated to the millions of
formal and informal caregivers around the world.

Table of Contents

About the Author

Patti Greene holds a Bachelor of Arts from Baylor University and pursued graduate studies at Southwestern Baptist Theological Seminary and the University of Missouri. She formerly served as a stay-at-home mother and school librarian before retiring to pursue her writing interests. She and her husband John have three children and five grandchildren. They currently live in Houston Texas. For the past few years, Patti and John have had the privilege of providing care to both Patti's mother and late father in her parents' home. Patti is also the author of three devotional prayer journals: *Awaken Me: Growing Deeper in Bible Study and Prayer* (2016), *Anchor Me: Laying a Foundation in Bible Study and Prayer* (2016) and *Answer Me: Developing a Heart for Prayer* (2016). When asked what she enjoys the most, she responds, "Ministry, no doubt about that!"

Preface

This book is all about caregiving. It is written for all caregivers—full-time caregivers, part-time, paid and unpaid, at home, at a distance, in a facility, and all others.

Caregivers around the world are responsible for caring and meeting the needs of those who are not able to care for themselves. The different roles they play in homes, medical facilities, and elderly housing communities are very important. Caregiving is a difficult job. Caregivers wear many hats such as housekeeper, menu planner, cook, driver, medication expert, health coordinator, and cleanliness facilitator. Some caregivers are professionally trained and certified in first-aid, cardiopulmonary resuscitation (CPR) and basic life support skills. Others are not, but they are just doing the best they can caring for a loved one either in a home or facility.

In this book, I have incorporated many topics associated with the task of caregiving. Whether one looks at it as an arduous task to complete or a God-given privilege, *Christian Caregiving* will provide practical advice for caring for your parents or loved ones. Both newcomers and veterans in the field will learn about the aging process, getting affairs in order, advocating, housing options, spirituality, and happily reaching the end of life. Beginners will be grateful for a short but informative introduction to multiple topics in one short read, and novices will be refreshed on the basic principles of being a compassionate provider. While this book is written mainly for family caregivers, those tending to the elderly in facility and home environments will gain valuable knowledge from the insights, tips, and Bible verses mentioned throughout this book.

It is this author's prayer that caregivers look at their caregiving responsibility as one chosen by God. For it is through Him that we acquire the strength, love, and joy to perform this job, vocation, or calling.

Chapter 1

Caregiving Basics

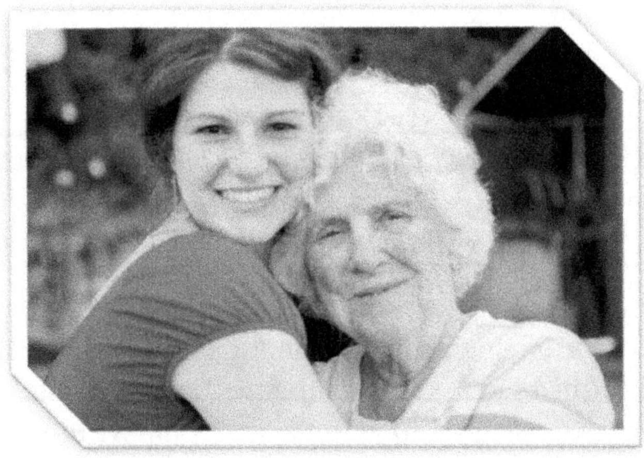

Photo 1. Grandmother and Granddaughter
by Dallas Totra (Lightstock)

There are many issues and facets involved in caring for ones' parents. The style and attitude of care, provided to a parent by a child, can vary considerably among the parent's children. One child embraces caregiving with a total outpouring of energy and love while another could experience a total depletion of energy and experience profound frustration. Still others could feel profound resentment at having this important responsibility 'dumped in their laps', either as a result of being out-maneuvered by other family members, or the one for whom it is most logical or practical to assume this role. In this concise book, the words *aged, elder, elderly, family member, loved one, parent, relative, senior,* and *senior citizen* are used interchangeably, as many people do care for other family members besides their parents.

The *Utah Caregiver Coalition* defines caregiving as "the provision of assistance to another person who is ill, disabled, or needs help with daily activities. It often requires attention to the physical, mental, social, and psychological needs and well-being of both the caregivers and the elderly person requiring care."[1]

In a Christian sense, caregiving is a call to serve and give your life to another person. Serving others is a theme discussed multiple times in the Bible as a virtue for us to strive for and act upon.

> ***Just as the Son of Man did not come to be served, but to serve, and to give His life a ransom for many.***
> ***(Matthew 20:28)***

In June Hunt's book *Caregiving: A Privilege, not a Prison,* she shares that caregiving provides emotional and physical support to someone unable to live independently and makes a choice with the heart and mind to give needed support to a dependent person. She also mentions that "Christian caregiving is offered in the spirit of love, compassion, and relationship."[2]

I was privileged to live with my mother and father during my father's final month of acute myeloid leukemia and dementia. Currently, my husband and I are living with my mother in her home as she faces her own critical health issues.

I strive for the same spirit Hunt describes as I face the many diverse issues relating to caring for my own mother as she embraces her final days, months, or years.

The Aging Process

Understanding how seniors age is a crucial issue. The elderly struggle with forfeiting their freedom and independence, becoming forgetful, losing their eyesight and hearing, experiencing mobility problems, encountering depression, and more. College degrees in aging address topics such as age-related diseases, the biology of aging, nutrition, laws, ethics of aging, and caregiving.

Your parents or loved ones may develop attitudes or thoughts they may never have had in their younger years. Feelings of loneliness, friendlessness, uselessness, and unwantedness may unfold. These feelings may show up as anti-socialness, depression, anxiety, or sadness. Issues such as living arrangements, financial matters, medical treatments, and legal issues may become household topics.

Too often caregivers have trouble adjusting to their parents' newfound attitudes and opinions. As their child, knowing your parents will help you understand why and how they act as they do. Facing these issues with a sound and patient mind will help your parents trust you and help them adjust to the uncertain future they—and you—are entering.

On the other hand, some seniors are even-keeled, sweet, sociable, and concerned with the welfare of others, all the while dealing with these important decisions; this helps make what could have been a difficult process much more manageable, and less stressful.

In the January 2017 issue of *Senior News*, an article titled, "When God Sends Help, Don't Ask Questions" looks at the case of an older woman who seemingly was very competent in coping with what life held for her.[3]

> She hurried to the pharmacy to pick up the medication. When she got back to the car, she found her keys locked inside.
>
> The woman found an old rusty coat hanger on the ground. She looked at it and said, "I don't know how to use this."
>
> She bowed her head and asked God to send her some help.

Within five minutes an old motorcycle pulled up, driven by a bearded man who was wearing an old biker skull rag. He got off his cycle and asked if he could help.

She said, "Yes, my husband is sick. I've locked my keys in my car. I must get home. Please, can you use this hanger to unlock my car?"

He said, Sure." He walked over to the car, and in less than a minute the car was open.

She hugged the man and through tears said, "Thank you, God, for sending me such a very nice man."

The man heard her little prayer and replied, "Lady I am not a nice man. I just got out of prison yesterday; I was in prison for car theft."

The woman hugged the man again, sobbing, "Oh, thank you, God! You even sent me a professional!"

Become Knowledgeable

In perusing the Internet, I found multiple tips on caregiving. They came under titles such as, *Tips for Caregivers; Caregiver Stress; Coping with Stress and Anxiety*. After immersing myself in these articles, and similar others, I have compiled a list of action items to help you get started with your caregiving *tour de force*:

- Get your parent's medical and legal information in order. Keep these items in a location easy for quick retrieval. The items and information you want to locate and secure include advance directives, wills, medication lists, birth certificates, insurance policies, estate planning documents, usernames, passwords, and safety deposit keys.
- Communicate with your parent's doctors, lawyers, pharmacists, and financial advisors.
- Find out what your loved one's preferences are regarding future living arrangements, long-term care, medical decisions, and legal issues while they can participate in these discussions themselves.

- Have candid conversations with your siblings. Delegate and plan a schedule for shared care even if one person is the primary caregiver.
- Understand that being your parent's caregiver is not an easy job. It is exhausting and possibly expensive, but it can be the most rewarding experience of your life.
- Understand that you are not alone. You may need to seek out support from others. Realize, however, that unless your friends or relatives have experienced caregiving themselves, they may not be capable of truly understanding your position.
- Watch for medical issues that may surface regarding your parents and yourself.

Be Proactive in Creating a Safe Environment

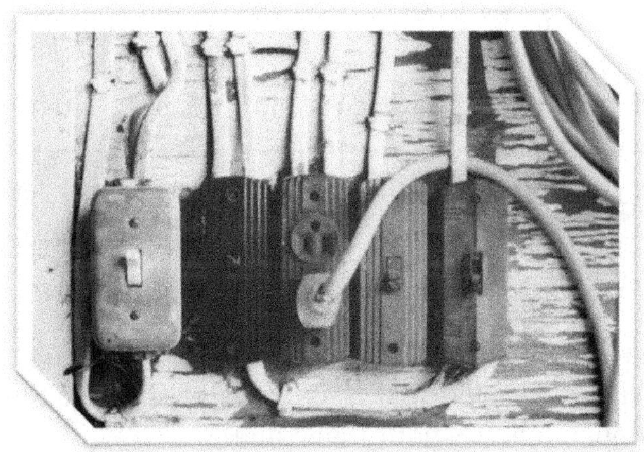

Photo 2. Vintage Power Outlets
by Brian A. Petersen (Lightstock)

Caregiving for your aging parents involves many aspects—especially caring for their safety.

Before addressing the safety of your parents, it is important to understand the aging process and to be knowledgeable about the issues facing the elderly. Then, it is time to become proactive regarding the safety issues facing your loved ones.

According to the U.S. Consumer Products Safety Commission (CPSC), "Many older Americans are injured in and around their homes every year. THE CPSC estimates that on average 1.4 million people aged 65 and older are treated in hospital and hospital emergency rooms each year for injuries associated with consumer products. Within this age group, the rate of injury is the highest for people 75 years of age and older."[3]

Too often caregivers are so overwhelmed with other critical issues that they overlook basic safety issues within the home. Some questions worth asking and answering about your parent's safety are:

- Are hallways free of clutter for walkers and wheelchairs?
- Are the rugs on the floor secure?
- Are the shelves in their living quarters secure?
- Are there flammable liquids around the house?
- Do you need to discuss fraud and scams, i.e. Internet fraud, telephone scams?
- Do you need to discuss not opening their doors to strangers?
- Do you need to discuss what to do in an emergency?
- Do you need to purchase a medical alert fall-protection system?
- Does the doorbell work?
- Have you identified home modifications to avert accidents, provide accessibility, and preserve the independence of your loved one?
- Will phone and electrical cords cause a tripping incident?
- Are your parents abusing alcohol or prescription drugs?

To familiarize yourself with more exhaustive home safety lists, it would be beneficial to peruse the Internet for some well-thought-out lists that may be specifically applicable to your loved ones' home and activities.

Driving

Many elderly men and women still drive. Some are capable; others are not. One of the hardest things any person must give up is their driver's license because it represents their independence and self-sufficiency. Caregivers must be actively involved in the driving safety of their loved ones. Sometimes adult children can tell their parents that it is time to relinquish their keys; other times it is best left up to a physician or other entity. Either way, securing the safety of your loved one and those around them is vital.

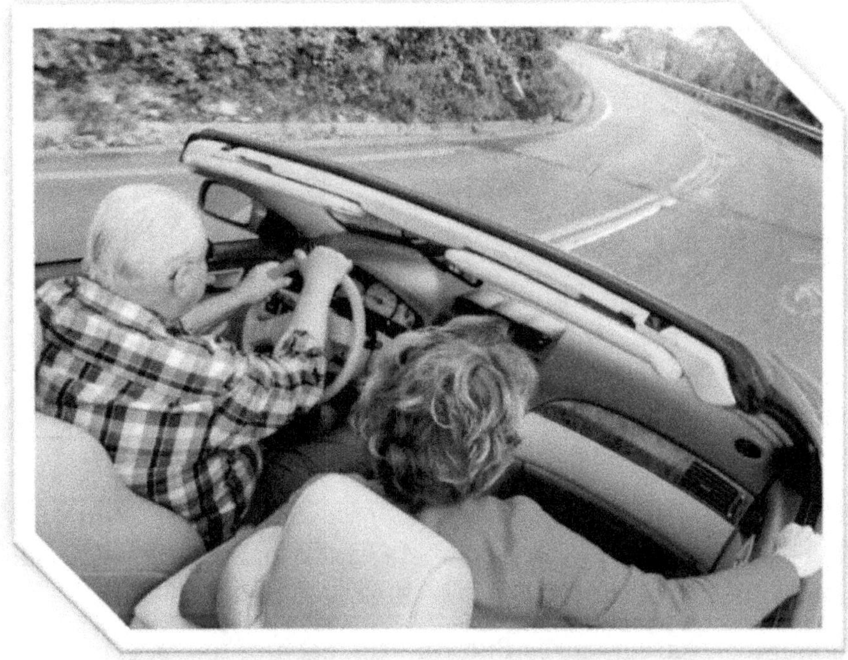

*Photo 3. An Elderly Couple Driving a Red Convertible
by Redman Creative (Lightstock)*

If your parents are still driving, some discussion questions to have with them include:

- Do you know not to drive when an emergency occurs?
- Do you know which routes are the safest to take?
- Have you had your hearing and vision checked recently?
- Is using a taxi, private driver, bus, or shuttle a possibility?
- Which is the best way to get to the doctor's office, home, church, grocery store, and other places?

There are many more exhaustive driving assessment checklists online that would be worthwhile for all caregivers to carefully examine.

Wrap Up

One of the most important things about caregiving is being informed. I was recently asked to teach a six-week class on "caregiving" at my church.

In preparing for the class I consulted many resources. I read books, websites, and articles on the topic. It was through learning more and listening to others that I felt better able to face the caregiving challenge with love and appreciation.

I was tasked with finding an appropriate book for the class. I bought and read multiple books and finally decided on the following resource—a very useful and instructive reference book on the topic of caregiving. I don't recommend books haphazardly, but this one is worth every penny!

Morris, Virginia. *How to Care for Aging Parents*, 3rd Edition: A One-Stop Resource for All Your Medical, Financial, Housing, and Emotional Issues. New York: Workman, 2014.

Remember, caregiving is different for each of us. As caregivers, we must learn more to understand the complexities of the aging process. By using various resources and becoming proactive in providing a safe environment for our loved ones or those assigned to our care, we can be assured we are providing for our own in a godly and honorable manner.

Bible Verses:

But if anyone does not provide for his own, and especially for those of his household, he has denied the faith and is worse than an unbeliever. (1 Timothy 5:8)

Rejoice always; pray without ceasing; in everything give thanks; for this is God's will for you in Christ Jesus. (1 Thessalonians 5:16-18)

Honor your father and your mother, as the LORD your God has commanded you, that your days may be prolonged and that it may go well with you on the land which the LORD your God gives you. (Deuteronomy 5:16)

Prayer:

Dear Lord, help me to be the best caregiver possible. Give me wisdom and a desire to honor You in how I serve. There are so many issues. You know my time and my schedule. Let me experience joy as I honor my loved ones. Let me seek knowledge. Let me be wise in my dealings with others. Let me be generous with my hugs and kisses. In Jesus' Name. Amen.

Chapter 2

Getting Affairs in Order

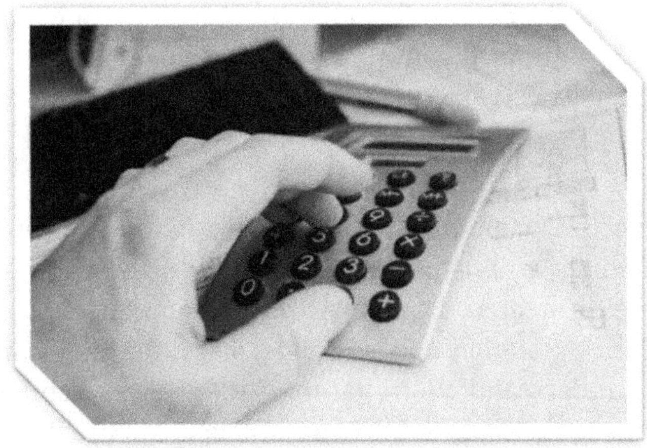

Photo 4. Using a Calculator
by Real Findo (Lightstock)

As a caregiver, one the most important things you can do for yourself and for your aging parents is to have a conversation with them about their legal, medical, financial, and personal affairs. It is often left up to the children to address these issues and "get the ball rolling" before a crisis occurs.

A story was told about three daughters who tried to have that talk with their mother, but she would always avoid the topic by steering the conversation in a different direction. Their 74-year-old mother then passed away unexpectedly after falling down a flight of stairs. Since "the conversation" never took place, they were left discovering their mother had a mortgage on her house. To complicate the matter, the bank which held the mortgage could not divulge any information to the daughters without a death certificate. The girls ended up finding important documents where they expected to find them: But then, they found their mother's insurance policy in a knitting bag![1]

Situations like this one create stress and frustration as offspring try to handle the affairs of others before and after their loved one's passing.

Many times, relatives can set their loved ones' affairs in order. Other times legal, medical, and financial help is needed to obtain the correct advice and documentation. Sometimes the three areas of legal, medical, and financial overlap, and other times an issue will fall directly into one category.

Legal

A legal specialty called "elder law" helps families locate specific help and advice to ensure an elder's estate, assets, and medical wishes are protected from possible upcoming legal, financial, and medical entanglements. An elder care attorney can usually help you understand your parent's information and situation more thoroughly. The result is an efficient approach to get you going in the right direction. Some families utilize their doctors, their financial advisers, and their own personal attorneys to reach the same goal. Different states have different laws and procedures for end-of-life planning, so it is always best to check what the laws are in your state, as some may require a witness, a notary signature, or an attorney signature.

No matter which route you choose, be proactive. With so many terms related to elder care planning, I have compiled the following list to guide you as you face the unique situations regarding your parents' affairs.

Legal Terms

It is essential to have an up-to-date will and/or trust that designates financial, estate, legal control, and distribution. You or the elder may have limited assets, but even with simple estates, it is generally advisable to have an attorney create a document that will protect the elder's wishes about his or her estate.

Many people confuse a *will* with a *trust*. While they both create designations for one's assets, *Elder Law Answers*, a long-term care and planning resource website, distinguishes the two by stating, "One main difference between a will and a trust is that a will goes into effect only after you die, while a trust takes effect as soon as you create it."

Will—A will is a document that directs who will receive your property at your death and it appoints a legal representative to carry out your wishes.

Trust—By contrast, a trust can be used to begin distributing property before death, at death or afterward. A trust is a legal arrangement through which one person (or an institution, such as a bank or law firm), called a "trustee," holds legal title to property for another person, called a "beneficiary." A trust usually has two types of beneficiaries —one set that receives income from the trust during their lives and another set that receives whatever is left over after the first set of beneficiaries dies."[2]

Durable Power of Attorney (DPOA)—A document that grants a person or persons ("Attorney-in-fact") the legal powers to perform on behalf of the elder ("Grantor") certain acts and functions specifically outlined in the document. This power is effective immediately and continues even if the grantor becomes disabled or incompetent. The powers usually granted include real estate, banking and financial transactions, personal and family maintenance, government benefits, estate trust, and beneficiary transactions.

Medical

As the elderly are living longer, caregivers have a longer period to oversee their parents. Therefore, it has become more necessary to understand the tenets of aging. The elderly tackle *aging gracefully* with chronic disorders, psychological or neurological issues, and physical limitations. The responsibility of seeking competent medical professionals, locating proficient healthcare agencies, and becoming proficient in medical forms and documentation is usually left to caregivers.

Medical Terms

Advance Directives—Written instructions regarding an individual's medical care preferences. The forms vary from state to state, but in general, advance directives can include a Living Will (not to be confused with a Last Will and Testament (will), a Healthcare Power of Attorney/Healthcare Proxy, a Do Not Resuscitate (DNR), a Do Not Intubate Order (DNI), and other documents. The National Institute on Aging defines an advance directive as "a legal document that goes into effect only if you are incapacitated and unable to speak for yourself." "Advance directives" are for people of all ages who might face any medical emergency or crisis. By maintaining up-to-date advance directives, you can be sure the medical treatment you want is carried out. It also relieves family members from making the gut-wrenching decisions that might occur in emergency situations. If you do not have any advance directives yet, it is advisable to start the process for you and your parents as soon as possible. It is not necessary to have a lawyer to create these medical documents. These documents should be kept in a handy, accessible location. For more information, The National Institute on Aging mentions many health resources and terms in their *Advance Care Planning* document.[3]

Living Will—A written document that notifies physicians how you want to be treated if you are dying or permanently unconscious and cannot make decisions about emergency treatment. [It is important to note that a living will is different from the legal will mentioned in the legal section above.]

Durable Power of Attorney for Health Care—A legal document naming a *healthcare proxy*, who is someone to make medical decisions for you at times when you might not be able to do so.

DNR (Do Not Resuscitate)—A document informing the medical staff in a hospital or nursing facility that you do not want them to try to return your heart to a normal rhythm if it stops or is beating unevenly. [Take this to the hospital and be sure your doctor has a copy of this document.]

DNI (Do Not Intubate)—A document that will alert emergency medical staff in a hospital or nursing facility that you do not want to be put on a breathing machine. [Take this to the hospital and be sure your doctor as a copy of this document.]

CPR (Cardiopulmonary Resuscitation)—Resuscitation that might restore your heartbeat when or if your heart stops beating or there is an abnormal rhythm in an emergency.

Ventilator Use—Ventilators are machines that help you to breathe by forcing air into your lungs. This tube, which is connected to the ventilator, is put through the throat into the trachea/windpipe. Putting the tube down the throat is called *intubation*.

Comfort Care—Comfort care is anything that can be done to soothe you and relieve suffering while staying in line with your wishes.

Artificial Nutrition or Artificial Hydration—When a person is unable to drink or feed themselves, a feeding tube and/or intravenous (IV) liquids enable the person to get their nutrition.

Palliative Care—A type of care focused on comforting patients with illnesses that are serious but not life-threatening for the time being. Its focus is to ease the pain and stress relating to serious and/or chronic illnesses. It is a multi-faceted/holistic approach to addressing physical, social, and spiritual needs of people dealing with illnesses such as kidney failure, congestive heart failure, and Alzheimer's.

Hospice Care—A type of care that provides comfort to you and your family during a life-threatening illness at the end of a person's life. It provides *care and comfort* to the patient and family rather than treatments to cure an illness (*palliative care*, see above). Hospice care is mainly for people who have less than 6 months to live and not likely to recover from their illness.

Organ and Tissue Donation—A donation allowing organs or body parts from a generally healthy person who has died to be transplanted into people who need them.

HIPAA (Health Insurance Portability and Accountability Act)—MedicineNet.com defines HIPAA as "a U.S. law designed to provide privacy standards to protect patients' medical records and other health information provided to health plans, doctors, hospitals and other healthcare providers."[4]

To have access to your loved one's medical records, written permission must be given. Doctors, hospitals, other providers of health care have HIPAA release forms for their patients to sign. These release forms authorize all or some medical information to be disclosed to other individuals or organizations. Checking to be sure you have access to your loved one's medical records is important. More information on medical advocacy may be found in Chapter 3.

Financial

The time may come when the elderly parent is not able to handle their own finances. This could be due to mental or physical impairment, visual difficulties, falling prey to scams, or the death of a spouse who handled the finances. Don't be afraid to step in to be sure financial losses do not occur. With the advent of computers, the elderly may easily transfer money, buy or sell stocks, or give money away without a family member even knowing. You may need to assess the situation and find out what tools will help prevent unfortunate situations from occurring.

Financial Terms

In the legal encyclopedia NOLO, Kathleen Michon defines the major financial terms family members should be familiar with.[5]

Joint Accounts—The elder can add you or another person to their checking account as a joint account holder. This makes both people a joint owner of the funds. Both can withdraw and deposit money and write checks. It allows the senior adult to maintain some independence and control and allows you to keep an eye on things, pay bills, and handle some (but not all) financial affairs.

Single-Owner Accounts with an Authorized Signer—A senior adult can add you as an authorized signer on a checking or savings account, without making you a joint owner. This means you can write checks and withdraw and deposit funds. However, because you are not an owner of the account, all transactions must be made on behalf of the senior adult.

Automatic Payments—You can ease the bill-paying burden by helping your loved one set up electronic automatic payments or withdrawals for monthly bills.

Representative Payee for Social Security Benefits—The senior adult can designate you as their representative payee for Social Security benefits. A representative payee receives the Social Security benefit checks and is responsible for using the funds on behalf of the elder.

Financial Power of Attorney—With a financial power of attorney, the senior adult gives another person legal authority to act on their behalf.

In addition, if your loved one has an Individual Retirement Account (IRA), stocks, mutual funds, or other accounts with financial institutions, a call to those businesses might be in order. They will be able to direct you as to handling the daunting situation you may be facing with your parents' financial matters.

More information on caregiving (including legal, medical, and financial) can be found at *The Caregiver's Handbook* at www.pbs.org/wgbh/caringforyourparents/handbook.[6]

For a list of essential documentation and information to gather and/or know where to locate before a person passes away, see Appendix 1.

Wrap Up

Let's face it: you may not feel equipped to initiate a conversation about the legal, medical, and financial decisions that you may encounter. But, when we approach our elders with kindness, listen to their opinions, and let them know that we are on their side to help them to make these decisions, we can proceed with confidence that we are carrying out their desires. The apostle Paul summed it up accurately when he writes:

> *Honor your father and mother. This is the first of God's Ten Commandments that ends with a promise. And this is the promise: that if you honor your father and mother, yours will be a long life, full of blessing.*
> *(Ephesians 6:2-3 LB)*

Bible Verses:

The King will answer and say to them, 'Truly I say to you, to the extent that you did it to one of these brothers of Mine, even the least of them, you did it to Me." (Matthew 25:40)

The Lord's bond-servant must not be quarrelsome, but be kind to all, able to teach, patient when wronged. (2 Timothy 2:24)

Bear one another's burdens, and thereby fulfill the law of Christ. (Galatians 6:2)

Prayer:

Lord, thank You for the many resources where I can find information to help me with my parent's legal, medical, and financial needs. Make me aware of information that is pertinent to the care of my parents. I truly want to be the best caregiver I can be. I need Your guidance and help. Let me love like You loved. Let me serve like You served. In Jesus' Name. Amen.

Chapter 3

Being an Advocate

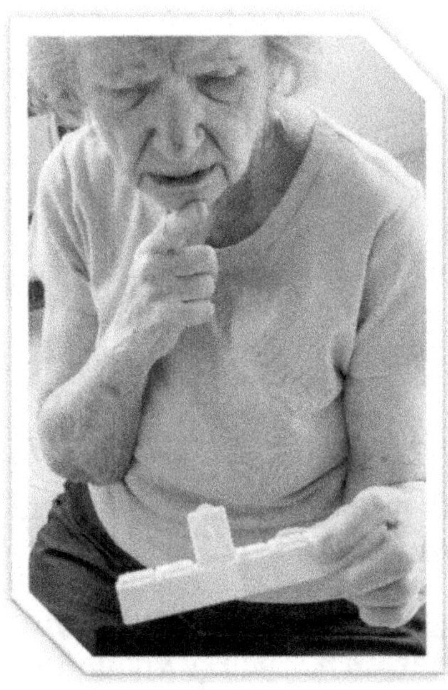

Photo 5. Elderly Woman Looking at Her Pill Box
by Jennifer Ruch (Lightstock)

The privileged or upper class can hire a personal healthcare advocate to help them with the issues they or their parents face as they age. Often the working class and middle class need to handle advocacy issues themselves or have their family members involved. Either way, all advocates need help with access to medication, transportation, and other individual challenges.

Advocacy

The *Merriam-Webster Dictionary* defines an *advocate* as "one who pleads the cause of others ."[1] Advocates speak up for "their client" when they can't speak up for themselves. While it would be nice for every elderly person to have their own personal healthcare advocate, it is usually left up to family members to advocate on behalf of their relatives rather than employing a paid staff member to help them navigate through the health and medical systems.

Your parents need you and their family members to:

- Be there to sign permissions
- Become familiar with their rights
- Resolve and discuss issues related to their health care
- Understand the intricacies of the services available
- Work on their behalf

Advocacy is essential when your parents reach a certain stage in life where they are unable to keep up with the complexities of the healthcare system. The elderly's main health advocacy topics revolve around their doctor visits, medication, illnesses and disorders, and dementia/Alzheimer's Disease.

> ***When they bring you before the synagogues and the rulers and the authorities, do not worry about how or what you are to speak in your defense, or what you are to say; for the Holy Spirit will teach you in that very hour what you ought to say.***
> ***(Luke 12:11-12)***

Medical—Doctor Visits

If possible, you or a family member should accompany the elderly to their doctor appointments. This is especially important if your parents have any cognitive disabilities. Establishing a relationship with your parents' doctors and the physician's office is the beginning of establishing an agreed-upon working plan for their health care.

Writing down questions for the doctor before the visit is always a good idea. No matter how trivial a question might seem to you or your parents, it is important to bring it up, so the doctor can piece together the entire picture, so the best care is given. However, keep in mind doctors only have so much time allotted for your visit, so prioritize your questions and comments to each physician.

Always bring a list of your parent's current medications to all doctor's appointments. Medications or dosages may change from week to week, so it is critical to inform every physician of all changes to vitamins, prescription drugs, and over-the-counter medicines. In addition, depending on your parent's insurance policies, you may want to ask your doctor to prescribe the generic medicine if it works as well as the non-generic.

After your visit, keep a record of what the doctor said, fill any new prescriptions, talk about the visit with your parents, and write down the next appointment date in your calendar along with a reminder to call for the results of any blood work.

Many physicians nowadays use a *portal*, a Web site which facilitates the two-way online collection and sharing of a patient's personal and health information between the doctor's office and the patient. Over the Internet, the patient may not only keep appointment and contact information up to date, and send/receive email, but view medical records such as doctor's notes and blood work results. Each physician may have his own portal, or several may share the same one; be sure to get your parent's username and password for each portal used by your parent's doctors.

Medications

Many seniors take an agglomeration of medication. It is a daunting task for them and their caregivers to make sure all medications are labeled correctly and administered properly. Care should also be taken to be sure your loved one is not using outdated medicine.

My mother has a medicine that comes in two dosages. The problem is that the pills are shaped the same; they are even the same size. One day my mother wasn't feeling well, and she noticed an irregular heartbeat. After a little detective work, we discovered she was taking a double dose of medicine because the two pills looked so similar except for the small numbered inscription on one side of the pill. It was quite evident that this double dose was causing a significant problem for her—one that was easily remedied but not always easy to detect.

Most adults over 65 years old take four or more medicines and monitoring them becomes very difficult. Using the same pharmacy for all prescriptions is advantageous and advisable. The pharmacist will have records of all the medicines taken and whether there are possible side effects and interactions with other medications. Once prescriptions are received, note the ailment that the prescription is prescribed for on the bottle or tube. Doing so will not only help you, but it will be extremely useful for anyone who might need to take over the elderly's distribution of medicine.

If your parents are not capable of handling their medications, it may be left up to an advocate, the caregiver, or you to manage them. Determining who will take on the responsibility for doling out, organizing, and storing their medicine is a major decision.

Illnesses and Disorders (Not Exhaustive)

The aged are living longer now than in previous generations. It follows, then, that as they live into their 80s, 90s, or even their 100s they will encounter a multitude of diseases and disorders. The most common issues affecting seniors, outside of accidents, are listed below:

- Blood
- Bone, joint, and muscle
- Brain, spinal cord, and nerve
- Cancer
- Digestive

- Ears, nose, and throat
- Eye
- Health issues and disorders of the elderly
- Hearing
- Heart and blood vessel
- Hormonal
- Immune
- Infections
- Injuries
- Kidney and urinary tract
- Liver and gallbladder
- Lung and airway
- Men's health issues
- Mental health
- Mouth and dental
- Nutrition and metabolic
- Skin
- Women's health issues

As an advocate for your parents, you must be aware and understand their condition(s). It is not uncommon for the elderly to fear telling you about new or reoccurring symptoms. They may be concerned about bothering you or they may be justly concerned that you might move them from their home to a facility if it appears they have too many problems. By telling them you are concerned and asking them to be honest with you, they are more apt to mention any symptoms they notice.

Unfortunately, if your parents are having memory problems, their ability to tell you about new symptoms may be diminished.

Dementia and Alzheimer's Disease

As we age, nothing is certain. No one knows what illnesses, if any, may be bestowed on them. But, one of the most devastating diagnoses imaginable is when you and your parents hear the words *dementia* or *Alzheimer's*!

The terms *dementia and Alzheimer's* are often used synonymously and interchangeably to represent changes in the brain which negatively affect cognitive function. However, Alzheimer's Disease is just one form of dementia. Other illnesses under the umbrella of dementia are Vascular Dementia, Dementia with Lewy Bodies, Mixed Dementia, Parkinson's Disease, Frontotemporal Dementia, Huntington's Disease, Normal Pressure Hydrocephalus, and Creutzfeldt-Jakob Disease.

The Alzheimer Foundation of America defines *Alzheimer's disease* as "a progressive, degenerative disorder that attacks the brain's nerve cells, or neurons, resulting in loss of memory, thinking and language skills, and behavioral changes." This foundation also describes *dementia* as "a general term for a decline in mental ability severe enough to interfere with daily life. Memory loss is an example. Alzheimer's is the most common type of dementia."[2]

When memory issued surfaced in one elderly lady, her children noticed a large quantity of cash being misplaced and eventually lost. In addition, her calls to her children were becoming much more frequent—many times a day. Matters like this may be the result of a declining memory; therefore, recognizing them as such is the first step in addressing these types of issues.

The signs were already there with my father. My mother and I noticed symptoms getting progressively worse over the years. His confusion, inability to calculate a tip, a slower reaction time, and forgetfulness became more pronounced as each season passed. By the time we took my father to a neurologist, we knew he had some form of dementia. When my father heard the word "dementia," his reaction was mixed. Mostly, he became worried about living and being a burden to his family, but at the same time, he was happy to put a name in conjunction with his symptoms. Everybody reacts differently to a "possible dementia diagnosis" or an "outright diagnosis." And, with dementia, your parents may react differently from day to day!

Speaking specifically to Alzheimer's disease, there are changes to the brain that have specific symptoms. While the symptoms vary from one person to the next, the National Institute on Aging mentions some of the most common initial symptoms of Alzheimer's disease:[3]

- Changes in personality
- Difficulty with word-finding
- Getting lost
- Impaired reasoning or judgment
- Vision/spatial issues

Since Alzheimer's is a progressive disease, once you notice memory and cognitive changes with your loved one, it is time to make an appointment with a neurologist. A neurologist will be able to discuss their symptoms with you. The physician will ask about the overall health of your parents, give memory tests, look at blood work, and possibly perform a CT, MRI, or PET scan to obtain a probable diagnosis. It is important to realize that other medical conditions can cause the same symptoms as dementia or Alzheimer's and the physician will want to rule those out so they can be addressed, i.e. brain tumors, thyroid disease, vitamin B12 deficiency.

Owen Darnell has written a beautiful Alzheimer's poem titled *Do Not Ask Me to Remember*.[4]

> Do not ask me to remember,
> Don't try to make me understand.
> Let me rest and know you're with me,
> Kiss my cheek and hold my hand.
> I'm confused beyond your concept.
> I am sad and sick and lost.
> All I know is that I need you
> To be with me at all cost.
> Do not lose your patience with me.
> Do not scold or curse or cry.
> I can't help the way I'm acting.
> Can't be different though I try.

Just remember that I need you.
That the best of me is gone,
Please don't fail to stand beside me,
Love me 'til my life is done.
And love says it all ...

> *Love is patient, love is kind and is not jealous; love does not brag and is not arrogant, does not act unbecomingly; it does not seek its own, is not provoked, does not take into account a wrong suffered, does not rejoice in unrighteousness, but rejoices with the truth; bears all things, believes all things, hopes all things, endures all things.*
> *(1 Corinthians 13:4-7)*

Government Assistance

Keeping up with the benefits and changes in Medicare or Medicaid is important because it can affect your loved ones' premiums, deductibles, hospital care, drug coverage and more. It is important not to miss deadlines for signing up and/or making changes that will affect your parent's coverage.

There may be changes for both Medicare and Medicaid under new and different government administrations. Reform is always in the works. Being vigilant and knowledgeable of these changes can affect the health and care of your parents.

As your parent's caregiver, overseeing their Medicare or Medicaid is vital.

Medicare

Medicare is the leading health insurance for people 65 or older. People under 65 with certain disabilities and people of any age with End-Stage Renal Disease (ESRD)— a permanent kidney failure requiring dialysis or a kidney transplant—are also eligible under the Medicare system.

A quick overview of Medicare from *What Medicare Covers* states,

Medicare Part A helps covers hospital insurance. In general, it covers hospital care, skilled nursing facility care, nursing home care, hospice, and home health services.

Medicare Part B helps cover medical insurance regarding medically necessary services and preventive services, such as clinical research, ambulance services, durable medical equipment, mental health, getting a second opinion before surgery, and limited outpatient prescription drugs.

Part A and B have premiums and out-of-pocket expenses which vary depending on personal factors.

Medicare Part C is a Medicare Advantage Plan that includes all benefits and services under Part A and B and more. The plan is provided by private companies, such as HMO's, PPO's, or PFFS (Private Fee for Service). Most plans under Medicare Part C have "copayments or coinsurance" and benefits. For these services and benefits, costs will vary.

Medicare Part D helps cover the cost of prescription drugs. Various prescription drug plans are run by private companies that are approved by Medicare. Costs, covered drugs, and premiums vary among plans.

Medigap (Medicare Supplement Insurance) is a private type of medical insurance that works with Medicare to assist with various out-of-pocket expenses such as, coinsurance, copayments, and other costs.[5]

For more information on Medicare, go to Medicare.gov.

Medicaid is a joint federal-state system providing health insurance to those requiring financial assistance. People must meet financial criteria to qualify for this public health insurance program. Medicaid is based on income. In the United States, low-incomed children, pregnant women, adults with dependent children, people with disabilities, and seniors are eligible for Medicaid. While every state established its own Medicaid eligibility, they must do so within the guidelines of the federal government.

Services Medicaid offers include physician and hospital visits, dental and vision services, and health screenings that are deemed *medically necessary.*

For more information on Medicaid, go to Medicaid.gov.

Caring for Yourself

Most caregivers are hesitant to talk about the needs they have while caregiving—the need for a break, for solitude, to be with their own friends, for respites, to be thanked and appreciated, and for additional finances. The list could go on, but these are some obvious needs for the caregivers/family members who have taken on the sole or close-to-sole responsibility of caring for a loved one. Some people are not emotionally or physically strong enough to consider full-time care of their parents, whether in a facility or in a home. Those situations should be respected. Everyone is different and has a different threshold. Thought should be given as to whom is best suited to take on the main caregiver role. Every family (including your loved one, if capable) must make some tough decisions regarding care. Family members should be held accountable to be a part of their parent's care. Siblings and other relatives should treat each other with respect and communicate what they can and cannot do to help. Full-time caregiving is time-consuming, physically demanding, and can be emotionally draining. Caretakers must take care of themselves before a critical burnout occurs.

Wrap Up

Advocating for your loved ones can be exhausting and over-whelming. Your spiritual life can be a real comfort during this season. Acting in Christian love will enhance your character and provide a renewed hope for your parents. Some days will be more trying than others. Praying to be the sons and daughters your parents need will give you strength and will help you to set a loving tone each day as you handle the infinite issues involved in your parent's care.

Your parents need you to help them manage and advocate for them through their doctor visits, medication challenges, illnesses, and insurance programs. Concentrate on short-term goals. Proceed one day at a time, never be afraid to seek a second opinion, and keep yourself healthy and stable.

Bible Verses:

So do not worry about tomorrow; for tomorrow will care for itself. Each day has enough trouble of its own. (Matthew 6:34)

A joyful heart is good medicine, but a broken spirit dries up the bones. (Proverbs 17:22)

Be devoted to one another in brotherly love; give preference to one another in honor. (Romans 12:10)

Prayer:

My heavenly Father, I can get so overwhelmed with all the jobs involved in caregiving. You know I love my parents. You know I care, but I get tired. There is so much to do each day. Give me Your strength and wisdom as I face the challenges ahead. Let me wake each day with a renewed love for You and my loved ones. Let me live day by day in Your presence. These things I ask in Jesus' Name. Amen.

Chapter 4

Choosing a Housing Option

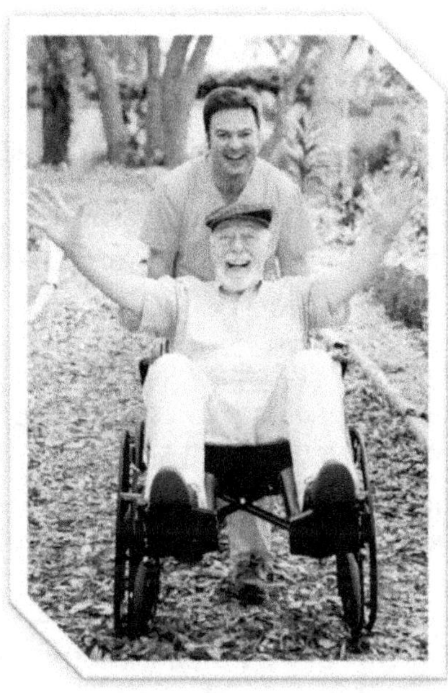

*Photo 6. Caring Nursing Home Orderly Pops a Wheelie
by Lisa F. Young (Shutterstock)*

Senior citizens are living longer. They have access to medical treatments which can prolong their lives. Thus, they are living longer compared to previous generations.

As a family caregiver, you will encounter complicated decisions regarding the living arrangements of your parents. While wanting to do the right thing, caregivers are often clueless about what housing options may be available. Below are a few *starter questions* to ask and ponder regarding your parents and their well-being.

Questions to Ask When Considering Housing Options

Safety Issues—Are your parents secure in their home? Is their driving safe for themselves and others? Are they able to take care of themselves?

Medical Issues—Are your parents able to administer and track their own medicine? What medical conditions do your parents have? Are they showing signs of memory problems?

Social Issues—Are your parents lonely? Do your parents have friends they like to socialize with?

Location—Are your parents happy where they live now? How will changing their current living situation affect them?

Cost—Are your parents financially able to sustain a decent standard of living? Are they able to afford their current housing arrangement?

Many parents are making cross-country migrations, leaving home to live with or be close to their children. In a *Chicago Tribune* article by Barbara Brotman, 93-year-old Elizabeth Larson tells a tender story about her move from Champaign, Illinois to be near her son, who lives in Hinsdale, Illinois.

> My son said that if anything happened, if I needed him, he was too far away, she said. She thought he was right. And she knew the solution, and that it would involve her leaving Champaign. Larson was sorry to leave neighbors she liked. But she didn't have to leave her two closest friends. They had already moved to "out-of-state retirement" complexes near their own adult children. So, it was easier for me to move, she said. And in a way, it was kind of exciting. I thought it would be nice to be near my son.[1]

While it was a nice amicable move for Elizabeth, it can be a gut-wrenching decision for others searching for senior housing options. Moving is a complex and confusing decision. The sooner you assess your parents' desires and needs, the sooner they can be in a living situation which they find more comfortable, practical, and pleasing. By becoming aware of the different housing options available, you may be the biggest asset in helping your parents come to terms with their living arrangement. The most common housing options are listed below. Discuss these options with your loved ones and give them time to consider what's best for them. Be kind, gentle, and patient as they face one of the most difficult decisions of their lives.

Housing Terms

Independent Care—Single or family living consisting of townhomes or apartments for self-sufficient seniors. They offer security and social activities in their community living setting. Services such as laundry, meals, transportation and social activities are usually provided. They are not regulated by the government. Independent Care facilities have a country club environment. The average cost to rent or buy a home, including community fees, can be up to $2,000 or more per month or more. They are also called *retirement communities, retirement homes*, or *senior apartments*.

Assisted Living—A community which provides 24-hour assistance. The personnel assist with eating, bathing and bathroom use. However, 24-hour medical service is not provided. Their care usually includes laundry, meals, transportation, social activities, toilet care, housekeeping, and medication aid. Assisted living communities are regulated by the state. Other names for assisted living facilities are *personal care homes, eldercare facilities, residential care facilities, group homes*, and *community residences*. The cost ranges from approximately $2,300-$5,500 per month.

Nursing Home—A community which provides 24-hour assistance with daily living and medical care by nurses and therapists. Nursing homes include doctors on call, hospice and end-of-life services, medication aid, housekeeping, toilet care, bathing, dressing, transportation, and laundry. Nursing homes adhere to both state and federal regulations. They are also called *rest homes, convalescent homes*, and *skilled nursing facilities*. The cost averages between $4,000-$12,000 per month.

Continuing Care Retirement Communities (CCRC)— *Continuing Care Retirement Communities*

Continuing Care Retirement Communities are retirement communities with housing accommodations for: independent living, assisted living, and nursing home care. CCRCs offer residents a continuum of care. A person can spend the rest of his/her lifetime in a CCRC, transferring between levels of care as needed. CCRCs have some state regulations. These facilities are also called *Continuing Care Retirement facilities* and *life care facilities.* Services and costs vary depending on the level of facility in which one resides. As with all facilities, checking the entrance fees and reading the residential agreement is very important.

Aging in Place—Many seniors decide to age in place. This is a living arrangement where the elderly and their children have made the choice to live in either the children's home, their parents' home, or the home of their choice for as long as they are capable. When assistance is needed, nurses, private aides, physical therapists, and other needed personnel will come to the home. Many seniors need to remodel their homes to make them suitable to meet their needs as they age.

Types of Care

Knowing what type of care your loved ones need narrows down the above housing options. *Assisted Living*, a premier publishing resource focused on providing high quality, trustworthy information about various aspects of senior living, gives some easy-to-understand definitions on the types of care available for the elderly population.3

Skilled Care—a type of intermediate care where the patient or resident needs more assistance than usual, generally from licensed nursing personnel and certified nursing assistants. This care is not the same as *long-term care,* in which a resident may not need the services of a licensed nurse daily.

Custodial Care—the type of care provided when seniors need paid caregivers or unpaid family caregivers to help look after them. Unfortunately, many older adults reach a time in their life when they can no longer care for themselves. They cannot get around the house without assistance. They cannot do the things they once did, as their physical and mental skills are not quite as sharp as they used to be. A caregiver may make all the difference for an older adult struggling with life's demands. The caregivers' helping hands can make an enormous difference in the elderly person's quality of life.

Palliative Care—Simply speaking, palliative care focuses on making a person feel better. It is a specific type of care that provides relief from: physical pain, chronic symptoms, and stresses related to their chronic or terminal illness. Nurses lend support to the patient and family, manage the pain, and improve the quality of life to a serious, chronic, and/or terminal patient. Palliative care usually occurs in a facility such as a hospital, assisted care facility, or nursing home that is associated with a palliative care team.

Hospice Care— Hospice is not a place; it is a concept. Hospice care most often occurs in a home environment. A hospice team consists of doctors, nurses, social workers, spiritual personnel, therapists, aides, and volunteers. Hospice does not focus on curing medical problems; rather, it centers on keeping the elderly pain-free, comfortable and happy (*palliative care*, see above) during their last days. In the *Hospice Handbook*, Larry Beresford says, "While hospice is care for the dying, it places special emphasis on life and living each day as fully as possible."[4] As mentioned earlier, eligibility in most hospice programs require an estimated death within the next six months due to the terminality of the patient's illness.

In *Knowing the Difference Between Hospice and Palliative Care*, journalist Susan Barton summarizes the difference between palliative care and hospice care as:

Palliative care provides comfort and controls symptoms for people who are dealing with a serious illness. Hospice care is palliative care for people whose life expectancy is limited. Understanding this distinction helps ensure you and your loved ones receive the right care.[5]

Home Care—a type of medical and assisted living in which the care provider works with the patient within their own home. Typically, the process involves an initial meeting between the care provider and patient to determine the personal needs and the level of care required. The care provider and patient will then come up with a personal and customized program to make sure the patient's needs are being met. The healthcare provider may be either a licensed professional or a part of a company which specializes in assisted living. Assisted living organizations are usually comprised of nurses, doctors, and other medical professionals who are assigned to each patient based on the patient's specific needs.

Residential Care Homes—A non-medical facility that provides room, board, housekeeping, personal care, and supervision in a home within a neighborhood community. Some residential care homes provide for specific types of residents experiencing; i.e. disabilities, mental issues, dementia. Residential care homes tend to be a good choice for seniors who are hindered in their ability to live independently or to be accepted into assisted living facilities. In most homes, residents have their own single room and live in a home atmosphere. The costs—usually half the price of nursing home care—vary and is usually paid by family or the residents themselves. In some areas, residential care homes are the last resort in terms of finding placement for residents who don't quite meet the criteria for nursing home care but may not have the funds for assisted living.

Adult Day Care—places senior citizens into the hands of licensed professionals who are fully capable of taking care of them during the daytime hours; these arrangements are analogous to those used by parents to tend to their small children while the parents are employed at work. For many people, this is a way for the elderly to get out of the house and socialize with other people. Socialization is extremely important; some people could easily slip into depression if they don't have someone they can talk to.

Companion Care—Companions for the elderly. Companion care personnel are usually trained by their company in safety and CPR. They are also called comfort caregivers. No certification is required to be a companion.

Due to different policies, it is important to consult with your physicians about what type of care is best for your parents.

When looking for a good care facility for your loved one, do your homework. Possible qualities to look for in a facility are positive reviews, acceptable residential agreements, qualified and happy staff, social programs, security, and emergency medical availability.

Paying for Housing

Often finding housing for our parents boils down to the financial ability to pay for services. Many seniors struggle with paying for their living arrangements as they age. Money runs out for some while others have difficulty managing their finances properly making it almost impossible to know what they can or cannot afford. Some ways to finance parental care are to use private savings from the parents or children, money from the sale of a home, long-term insurance, reverse mortgages, Medicare or Medicaid, VA benefits, stocks/bonds, non-profit organizations, or private organizations.

As family members face the prospect of caring for their aging parents, complex decisions about housing are imperative. Each housing option listed above comes with benefits and complexities. It is up to the family to educate themselves on what is available by communicating with representatives of these housing and care choices and set aside time to formulate a plan that works for you and your parents.

The *Paying for Senior Care* website assists individuals in the planning and implementing of long-term senior care. This website discusses how financial planning is a must to handle *aging in place* and for providing money for private and public financial care in assisting you with this task of long term care.[2]

Wrap Up

When my father passed away, my husband and I decided to move into my mother's home to care for her on a full-time basis. It was a mutual decision on our parts with the understanding that we would talk if the situation was not working well for any of us. As retired baby boomers, our situation allowed this arrangement. While it isn't for everybody, the decision was a joint one, made in the best interest of both my mother and ourselves.

As you face upcoming living arrangements for your parents, be open-minded, respectful, realistic, and informed.

> *Honor your father and your mother,*
> *that your days may be prolonged in the land*
> *which the LORD your God gives you.*
> *(Exodus 20:12)*

The expression "there's no place like home" is true. But, when the time comes when parents need to consider whether to move or not, let's make sure that whatever plan is crafted creates a secure, comfortable and pleasing environment for all involved.

Bible Verses:

Whoever speaks, is to do so as one who is speaking the utterances of God; whoever serves is to do so as one who is serving by the strength which God supplies; so that in all things God may be glorified through Jesus Christ, to whom belongs the glory and dominion forever and ever. Amen. (1 Peter 4:11)

Cease *striving* and know that I am God. (Psalm 46:10a)

Therefore, having been justified by faith, we have peace with God through our Lord Jesus Christ. (Romans 5:1)

Prayer:

Dear Lord, As I face caring for my parents, please help me to honor and respect them in all decisions that must be made regarding living arrangements. I trust that You will guide me and give me wisdom as plans and decisions are made. Thank you, Lord, for helping me. In Jesus' Name. Amen.

Chapter 5

Facing Spiritual Issues

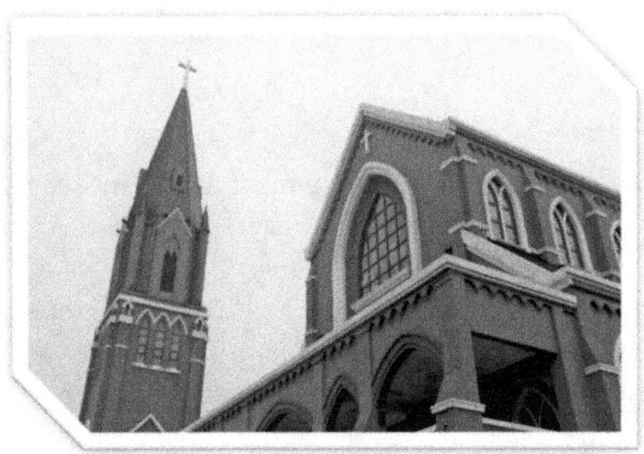

Photo 7. Traditional Church and Tower
by Rob Birkbeck (Lightstock)

My mother is 92 years old. Her health is extremely fragile, but her mind is remarkable and her memory is strong. Recently I drove my mother and her friend to their church for a special Women's Club luncheon and presentation. After the meal, many women lingered and chatted, laughed, and enjoyed fellowship together. You might ask why I chauffeur my mother around like this; I do it because I love my mother and I want her to continue to enjoy the church she has attended for the past 50 years. It is there she fellowships with her friends and shares a spiritual connection with others and the Lord.

As a caregiver, concerns usually center around the emotional, physical, and social lives of our loved ones. One aspect often lacking in caregiving is an interest in the elderly's spiritual life.

Whether you are a part-time caregiver or a full-time caregiver, giving yourself to the spiritual needs of your parents is truly a privilege.

For those who take their spirituality seriously, a sense of purpose and fulfillment undergirds their lives. Despite this fact, some do not understand or take seriously this component of another's life. Understanding spirituality is complicated because there are so many scenarios and so many definitions of spirituality at play. Your participation involves answering a few questions.

Questions to Ask Yourself

- Are you a part-time caregiver or a full-time caregiver?
- Are your parents living in the same town or city as you are?
- Are you a strong believer, a 'sort of' religious person, or an uninterested individual?
- Have your parents lived a dedicated life to God and the church?
- Have they attended church sporadically?
- Have they rarely explored any 'religious' life?

Once you mix and match all these different dynamics together, it is time to discern and pray about your part in your parents' spiritual life. Allowing your parents to pursue or continue their interests in God, church, and spiritual growth is an important part of regular caregiving. However, regardless of your or your parents' spiritual background, caring for them is one of the most compassionate undertakings you and your siblings can do.

Serving others is a privilege. Serving gives purpose in your own life, allows for God to use you, and may be the answer to someone else's prayers.

> *Be kind to one another, tender-hearted, forgiving each other, just as God in Christ also has forgiven you.*
> *(Ephesians 4:32)*

The Facts

Many seniors who have attended church all their lives develop a deeper desire for the things of God as they age. Others do not. Some seniors glide into old age making their spirituality more of an inward feat rather than a community effort. Some studies have concluded that one's interest in spiritual matters increases as one ages while others say the reverse.

Health care professionals who assess, treat, and work with the aged from middle to later life are called *gerontologists*—not to be confused with a *geriatrician* who is a medical doctor who specializes in treating the medical problems of the elderly, akin to a pediatrician who treats the medical conditions of children. Both gerontologists and geriatricians recognize how the spiritual life regarding their patients yields an unexplainable peace and calmness as the elderly face the future. As a result, their physical well-being is often affected in a positive way. They see their spiritually-minded clients and patients as possessing strength and tranquility regarding their future.

Why Seniors Renew or Deepen their Faith as They Age

- Concern about their death and the afterlife
- Concern over their reduced income, the ability to meet their needs, their health, and their family
- More time to pray and read their Bible
- Need strength as they face illnesses, loss of friends, and loneliness
- An inward desire from the Holy Spirit to strengthen their dependence on God

At a time when seniors tackle new challenges, many lose their support systems. This should be a huge consideration in churches as "baby boomers" start drifting into the senior adult category.

Why Seniors Abandon their Faith and Church

- Difficulty adjusting to change—The new programs and facilities are too much for them. Adjusting to change is especially hard for the aging population
- Hearing loss—They can't hear the preacher or Sunday school teacher
- Lack of activities for seniors—Feeling of alienation may occur when more emphasis is given to children ministries, youth ministries, young adult ministries, or any ministries besides senior adult ministries
- Miss traditions—They feel left out, unwanted, unneeded in the congregation. Seniors enjoy the familiarity of things past, i.e. hymns, Sunday dinners, fellowship luncheons
- Other disabilities—There may not be handicapped parking or wheelchair accommodations at the church. They may be unable to get to church due to disability or inability to drive themselves. Or maybe, there is too much walking to get to their classes or sanctuary.
- Sin—Disobedience to God's commandments and mandates
- Stimulating services (music, yelling, confusion)—In *Negative Noise and Alzheimer's*, Stanton O. Berg quotes the British Alzheimer's Society by stating that, "[People with Alzheimer's] feel bewildered or anxious because there is too much noise, too many people around, or a change in a familiar routine."[1]

Just as it is important to care for your loved ones' physical needs, it is paramount to be cognizant of your parents' spiritual needs as well.

Practical Ways You Can Help Your Loved Ones

- If you live in the same town or city as your parents, bring them to church and church functions.
- If you live out-of-town, contact their church organization, friends, or other family members to set up transportation.

- If you or family members live in the same city or town, be sure to visit them.
- If your parents are in a facility, investigate what kind of spiritual activities are available.
- Make their living environment familiar and comfortable, i.e. put their favorite cross in their room, be sure their Bible is easily accessible.
- Provide notecards, stamps, and addresses so they can write and minister to their friends.
- Purchase a large-print Bible for them if needed.
- Schedule an appointment with an audiologist to get their hearing checked.
- Schedule an appointment with an optometrist or an ophthalmologist to get their eyesight checked.

> *Whoever speaks, is to do so as one who is speaking the utterances of God; whoever serves is to do so as one who is serving by the strength which God supplies; so that in all things God may be glorified through Jesus Christ, to whom belongs the glory and dominion forever and ever. Amen.*
> *(1 Peter 4:11)*

Questions Caregivers Must Ask

Below are a few questions caregivers must ask. Spend some time thinking, meditating, and praying for additional questions that need to be asked and how you can be a part of the solution.

- What hindrances are my parents facing?
- My parents used to attend church. Why don't they go now?
- How do I approach my unbelieving parents about Jesus Christ?

What is Your Spiritual Condition?

Being connected to God's divine source can help you manage better as your caregiving duties progress. Continuing or starting to seek God's presence and strength in your life will assist you as you care for and minister to your loved ones. Understanding you are not perfect alleviates a mindset of inadequacy. Remind yourself of all your parents have done for you. If they haven't done much, it is time to ask God how He wants you to treat them and care for them regardless of the past. God is available to help you as you support your parents. By being their caregiver, you can be assured, God has given you a divine assignment—one that you won't regret.

One way to keep in touch with the Lord is to pray. As believers, praying should happen daily—especially when you are adjusting to a new phase in both your and your parents' lives. Listed below are ten tips for a better prayer life taken from my book, *Answer Me: Developing a Heart for Prayer.* I encourage you to read and meditate upon the thoughts and verses located in your Bible to help you during this caregiving season of life.

Ten Tips for a Better Prayer Life

1. Understand there is a scriptural basis for prayer.

> God specifically tells us to pray. The principle of 'calling on God' is mentioned multiple times in Scripture. The Bible tells us to pray explicitly and the LORD will answer our prayers and tells us great and hidden things not known. (Read Jeremiah 33:3)

2. Use a framework when praying.

> Prayer consists of many aspects—praise, worship, thanksgiving, confession, and petition. People from both the Old Testament and New Testaments prayed. Prayer unleashes the Holy Spirit and ignites a change in us. God's people and God's church are empowered through prayer. (Read Matthew 6:9-13)

3. Understand we are called to pray.

> Believers are called to pray. God can do whatever He wants to do, but He delights in working through our prayers. Praying takes discipline. It is our responsibility to pray for ourselves and for the needs of others. Some-

times we hesitate to pray because we do not believe that there will be results. (Read 1 Samuel 12:23)

4. Just ask.

God wants us to ask for what we need. The Bible mentions numerous things we can pray about for ourselves, such as good health, God's will, wisdom, and strength. Matthew 7:11 states, "If you then, being evil, know how to give good gifts to your children, how much more will your Father who is in heaven give good things to those who ask him!" (Read 2 Chronicles 1:11-12)

5. Be bold.

Be bold—do not be general or half-hearted in our requests to God. God wants us to be bold in our prayers. Ask the Lord for a verse to speak especially to us. Claim God's promises in prayer. (Read John 15:7, John 15:16, John 16:23-24, and Acts 4:31)

6. Pray the Scriptures.

Many people have discovered the power of praying Scriptures in their communication with God, thus developing confidence in their prayers. To "pray the Scriptures," try substituting names, pronouns, places, and circumstances into the Word of God. (Read Hebrews 4:12)

7. Agree in prayer.

Sometimes we pray with no results. This might be a time to call for others to pray with us. Jesus promises to be with us when two or more are gathered in His name. When united in prayer, God's power multiples as our prayers are uplifted and intertwined in the Holy Spirit. (Read Matthew 18:19-20)

8. Read the Bible in addition to praying.

2 Timothy 2:15 (KJV) says to, "Study to shew thyself approved unto God, a workman that needeth not to be ashamed, rightly dividing the word of truth." Spending time in Bible study and prayer causes our spirits to become sensitive to His leading. Succumbing to today's culture of liberalism is easy, but when the words of God

dwell within His people, we are less likely to be led astray. (Read James 1:5)

9. Believe in His divine providence.

The universe is not governed by fate. God is in control of every occurrence in the universe. All that happens is because it is either His will or He allowed it. Because God is involved in everything in the world, He can answer our prayers because He sees the "big picture" unfolding in our lives. (Read Psalm 103:19)

10. Pray for God's will.

While there is no set procedure for knowing God's will, His will never contradicts what His Word says. With Biblical guidance, prayer, counsel of mature believers, faith, glimpses from the Holy Spirit, and sometimes miraculous intervention, revelation of His will is possible. (Read Hebrews 11:8)[2]

Eternal Life

On our most recent visit to my mother's oncologist, we were discussing Mom's current and future prognosis. In his matter-of-fact intonation, he said, "Life is a terminal illness!" While we don't want to think about life like this, it is true. We all will die and face an eternal future.

As we live our earthly life, let us be ever mindful of our eternal destination. Gaining an understanding of our future existence is significant in understanding life-and-death anxieties and angsts.

Caregivers, parents, and all humanity will die. As already noted, many adults have a renewed interest in heaven as they age. CRU (formerly Campus Crusade for Christ) discusses four laws in the booklet "Have You Heard of the Four Spiritual Laws?"[3] It examines how people—people of all ages, young and old—can become Christ-followers.

Four Spiritual Laws

Law 1: God loves you and offers a wonderful plan for your life (John 3:16).

Law 2: Man is sinful and separated from God. Therefore, he cannot know and experience God's love and plan for his life (Romans 3:23).

Law 3: Jesus Christ is God's only provision for man's sin. Through Him, you can know and experience God's love and plan for your life (John 14:6).

Law 4: We must individually receive Jesus Christ as Savior and Lord; then we can know and experience God's love and plan for our lives (Revelation 3:20).

A Heart-to-Heart Prayer

Many seniors seek an assurance of heaven and are quite willing to talk to God and start depending on Him—even if they have not shown any interest in things of God in the past. Countless older adults renew their faith by consecrating or renewing their life to God. This one act brings peace, comfort, and eternal assurance as they face the rest of their life. A short prayer from one's heart—like the one below—may give that needed assurance to the souls of many "searching seniors."

Dear God, I know I'm a sinner, and I ask for Your forgiveness. I believe Jesus Christ is Your Son. I believe that He died for my sin and that You raised Him to life. I want to trust Him as my Savior and follow Him as Lord, from this day forward. Guide my life and help me to do Your will. I pray this in the name of Jesus. Amen.[4]

If you believe in God's gift of salvation, but your parents haven't, now is a good time to have a candid heart-to-heart with them. Share your life and testimony with them.

Eight days before my father passed away, I had a candid heart-to-heart with him. He prayed a prayer akin to the prayer written above. As we sat on his couch at 5 a.m., we quietly talked together and talked to God. Some may call this a "deathbed conversion". No matter what it is called, my father accepted Jesus Christ and God used me to help him make a decision that gave him peace and comfort to face the days ahead.

Wrap Up

Caretaking means being responsible for various aspects of your parents' life. As we face our parents' sundown years, let's do what we can to help them hold on to, delight in, and agree to take part in their spiritual life while at the same time progressing and preserving our own spirituality.

Bible Verses:

You shall rise up before the grayheaded and honor the aged, and you shall revere your God; I am the LORD. (Leviticus 19:32)

The LORD is my shepherd, I shall not want. He makes me lie down in green pastures; He leads me beside quiet waters. He restores my soul; He guides me in the paths of righteousness. For His name's sake. Even though I walk through the valley of the shadow of death, I fear no evil, for You are with me; Your rod and Your staff, they comfort me. You prepare a table before me in the presence of my enemies; You have anointed my head with oil; My cup overflows. Surely goodness and lovingkindness will follow me all the days of my life, And I will dwell in the house of the LORD forever. (Psalm 23:1-6)

Finally, brethren, rejoice, be made complete, be comforted, be like-minded, live in peace; and the God of love and peace will be with you. (2 Corinthians 13:11)

Prayer:

Dear heavenly Father, as I consider all the needs of my parents, let me be mindful of their whole being. I pray for their emotional, physical, social, and spiritual life. Make me aware of their needs. Let me offer my help. Give us both peace and comfort as we face the days ahead. In Jesus' Name. Amen.

Chapter 6

Navigating to "The Finish Line"

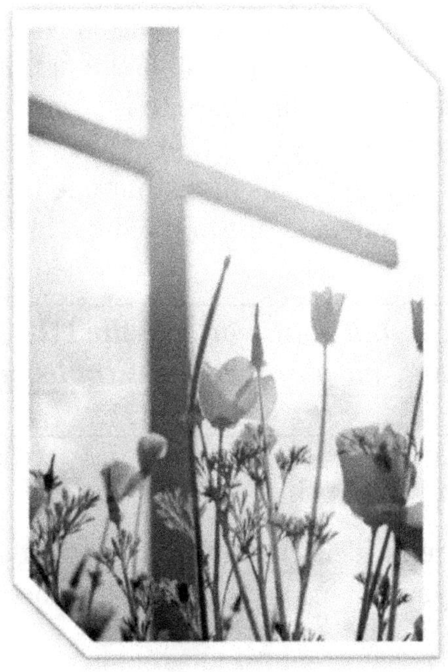

Photo 8. Flowers Growing Under a Cross Glowing in Sunlight
by Neely Wang (Lightstock)

Ask any recent mother about her child delivery experience and you will not hear the same run-of-the-mill story. Each woman's childbirth experience is different and personal.

As a point of comparison, there are just as many accounts about the dying process. Just as we come into this world in our own unique way, we will also leave it in our own distinctive fashion. But, one thing is for sure: We will all die! Our life story will be different than anyone else's story as evidenced by diverse obituaries and hand-me-down family stories.

We hate to admit it, but simply stated, death is a part of life.

One day your parents might be sitting on the couch chatting with you. A week or so later, they may be lying in bed struggling with labored breathing. You may be alarmed by the death rattle you hear in their chest. Shortly thereafter, they might die in your arms or while you are in a different room. But, then what?

When a loved one is close to passing, we will face impending pain, grief, and sadness—especially when that final moment occurs. Often, we wish we had time to rest, mourn, and cry right after the death of our loved ones—but we can't. We are thrust into dealing with the practical steps that need to be taken. Being prepared for this moment is one of the most important steps you can take.

> **Commit your works to the LORD.**
> **And your plans will be established.**
> **(Proverbs 16:3)**

Preparing for the Finish Line

If your loved one is lucid, having information available will be very helpful to you when the time of death occurs. Information may include:

- Decisions about organ donations, autopsies, and/or embalming are all good decisions to have made before your loved one passes away.
- Instructions pertaining to burial and funeral arrangements, pastoral information, favorite Bible verses or songs to use at the funeral.
- Location of important documents. Examples include the will, people to notify upon death, personal documents, debts, monthly expenses, keys and combinations to car, home, and safety deposit boxes, pension papers, bank account information, insurance information, Social Security

number, login credentials for all online accounts, business instructions, tax returns, valuable possessions, birth certificates, marriage certificates, car titles, insurance policies and retirement documents.

- Personal information such as, the names of colleges and degrees, certifications, past and current employers. This information is invaluable to those left behind for probate, obituaries, and other important duties that need to be carried out. (See Appendix, Table 1)

If a person has been disinherited from a will, obtaining a duly-authorized written record of the disinheritance will help in resolving any disputes or contesting of the will.

Signs that Death is Near

The *National Caregivers Library* website examines signs and symptoms that relate to the impending death of a loved one. Possible indicators suggest that as death becomes closer, you might notice that your parent might sleep more, be less verbal, eat less, drink less, encounter more pain, develop changes in blood pressure, experience a change in heart rate, undergo changes in skin, go to the bathroom less, become incontinent, suffer with confusion, experience erratic breathing, exhibit restlessness, endure difficulty swallowing, see visions, show evidence of glazed eyes, and extremities may appear bluish in color.

Saying Goodbye

Knowing when to call the family to say goodbye is difficult to gauge. When you notice symptoms, you may want to let family and close friends know so an opportunity to say a final farewell may occur. Obviously, at this point, you don't know the exact time that death will occur, but most loved ones would appreciate a "heads up!"[1]

It is interesting that many people before death have a moment of lucidity. It happened the night before my father passed away. All the family was standing around his bed. He opened his eyes, looked at everyone and gave the biggest grin ever. It was so remarkable that he knew and loved seeing his family around during his last hours combatting leukemia. After seeing us all, he clapped for us. What a memory to cherish!

Embracing the Final Moments

> *I will ask the Father, and He will give you another Helper,*
> *that He may be with you forever.*
> *(John 14:16)*

If death occurs in a hospital or facility, the staff will usually guide you as to the steps that must take place. If the death occurs at home under a hospice situation, there is no need to rush to call the funeral home.

Lingering around your loved one to say goodbye and comfort others is acceptable. When the hospice agency is called, they will support you and the family through your grief. They can also help you by contacting the designated funeral home if you have one. A death must be pronounced by a medical doctor or hospice nurse. Having hospice already in place will help the family during this difficult time.

It is worth mentioning that without hospice, the process will be more complicated. You will be responsible for making arrangement for your loved one to be picked up. But first, you will need to call 911. When an ambulance arrives, you might be asked when the time of death occurred. Be prepared to show a DNR (Do Not Resuscitate Order) especially if you have waited over an hour to call them.

> *There is an appointed time for everything.*
> *And there is a time for every event under heaven—*
> *A time to give birth and a time to die.*
> *(Ecclesiastes 3:1-2a)*

Let's be prepared for God's moment and His timing by being wise, fruitful, and loving while we embrace our loved ones' last days—in both the practical and spiritual sense.

After Death Occurs

Request Death Certificates

When my father passed away, the funeral home told us to request at least 20 copies of his death certificate. There will be many instances where you will need them as you clear up their estate, personal affairs, and business. If the funeral home you are using does not supply those to you, they can be obtained by contacting the Vital Statistics office in the state where the death occurred. Most organizations will require an original death certificate, not a copy.

Inform All Financial Establishments

After you receive the death certificates, it will be time to contact all institutions regarding the passing of your loved one. Insurance companies, credit card companies, mortgage companies, brokerage firms, and banks should be notified. Be aware that once banks are notified of a death, the accounts are usually frozen until new accounts are set up with the survivors; this may take longer than anticipated, so be sure the family has enough money to get by until this is taken care of.

Get in Touch with Providers

Contact utility companies (telephone, cable, Internet service providers) for cancellation or name changes. It is not imperative to cancel home services such as gas, water, electric, lawn services, pest control until a later date. This will ensure that the home or apartment can continue to be maintained until decisions are made.

Report the Death to Government Agencies

Notify the Social Security office and the Veteran's Administration about the loss of your loved one. While some benefits might be canceled, others may be adjusted for survivor benefits. If your parents were veterans, survivor benefits may be available depending on the eligibility for you or other family members.

Contact Employers and Former Employers

Contacting current or former employers is essential. The Human Resources departments of these organizations will help you sort out benefits, life insurance, stocks, and beneficiary information. By contacting former companies, you might be surprised to find out that there is a death benefit that you are unaware of. It is your responsibility to find out about that, not theirs![2]

Probate the Estate

The word "probate" or phrase "probating the will" is used many times after deaths. It is the legal process that takes place after someone dies to administer the deceased estate. If there is no will, each state has rules and lists of qualified individuals to help you with distribution. If the deceased had a will, there is usually an executor who is responsible for handling the distributing of wealth and property once a person dies. Having a will significantly simplifies the probating process. If you have been named an executor, you must show proof of your role before working in that capacity; this is usually stated in the person's will or an addendum. After one dies, all beneficiaries and heirs must be notified. An inventory must be taken of all the estate assets and creditors should be notified. All estate expenses, including funeral expenses, taxes, and debts must be paid from a person's estate. And finally, all legal property titles will be transferred and distributed according to the will. Depending on the deceased's estate, it can take up to a year or longer to sort out all the details.

Wrap Up

When your loved one dies, there are no easy answers or exact protocols to follow. There will be pain, grief, and sadness.

When the apostle Paul spoke of death, he said, "according to my earnest expectation and hope, that I will not be put to shame in anything, but that with all boldness, Christ will even now, as always, be exalted in my body, whether by life or by death" (Philippians 1:20).

We cannot trivialize death. We will miss our parents or family members when they die. It's easy to focus on ourselves and the loss that we have encountered both before and after they pass away. Many people who spent the days, weeks, and months before an impending death giving their loved ones' support, compassion, love, and care find that the memories of the last moments with their loved one very comforting. But, as we grieve the loss of our parents, let's remember that there is a time for everything—including death. The time was chosen by God; rest in this comforting thought.

> *There is an appointed time for everything. And there is a time*
> *for every event under heaven—*
> *A time to give birth and a time to die;*
> *A time to plant and a time to uproot what is planted.*
> *A time to kill and a time to heal;*
> *A time to tear down and a time to build up.*
> *A time to weep and a time to laugh;*
> *A time to mourn and a time to dance.*
> *A time to throw stones and a time to gather stones;*
> *A time to embrace and a time to shun embracing.*
> *A time to search and a time to give up as lost;*
> *A time to keep and a time to throw away.*
> *A time to tear apart and a time to sew together;*
> *A time to be silent and a time to speak.*
> *A time to love and a time to hate;*
> *A time for war and a time for peace.*
> *(Ecclesiastes 3:1-8)*

As we deal with the death of our family members, bear in mind that God knew when our loved one would be born and when they would die. Let's rest in the fact that God has known the "big picture" in their life just as He knows the "big picture" in our lives. Let's view this new season in life as the beginning, not the end—a time to exalt and glorify God. When we envision that our real home is in heaven, it may be a little easier to let our loved ones go. Best wishes.

Bible Verses:

Even though I walk through the valley of the shadow of death, I fear no evil, for You are with me; Your rod and Your staff, they comfort me. (Psalm 23:4)

But if any of you lacks wisdom, let him ask of God, who gives to all generously and without reproach, and it will be given to him. (James 1:5)

In my distress, I called upon the LORD, and cried to my God for help; He heard my voice out of His temple, and my cry for help before Him came into His ears. (Psalm 18:6)

Prayer:

Most gracious God. Please be with me as I face the final days of my loved one's life. Let me care for them as You care for me. I need Your wisdom, Your grace, and Your peace. I need You now more than ever during this time when decisions need to be made. Let me be pre-prepared—both physically, emotionally and spiritually to know Your will during this difficult time. In Jesus' Name. Amen.

Appendix: TABLE 1

Table 1. Essential Documentation to Initiate, Locate, and File for Your Elderly Parents

Legal	Medical	Financial	Personal	Contact Information
Attorney	Advance Directive Documents/Living Will	Bank Account Information	Home/Real Estate Holdings	Financial Advisor
Power of Attorney	Medical History	Safety Deposit Box and Keys	Keys/Combinations	Insurance Agent
Last Will and Testament	Prescriptions/Dosages	Stocks; Bonds, 401 (k)s	Birth Certificate	Bankers
Durable Power of Attorney	Healthcare Specialists	Annuities	Marriage Certificate	Attorney
Beneficiaries	Medical Power of Attorney	IRAs	Vehicle Information/Titles	Accountant/Tax Planner
Contracts		Mutual Funds	Social Security Card	Physicians
		Gold, Silver, Jewels, etc.	Retirement Records	Church/Pastor, Priest, Rabbi
		Life Insurance Policies	Utility Providers	Funeral Home
		Government Entities	Pet Information/Vet	Hospice Personnel
		Business Interests	Valuable Possessions	Home Healthcare Agency
		Account Numbers, and Digital Login Data	Money Owed	Beneficiaries
		All Investment Accounts	Memorial Instructions; Obituary Information	Credit Union
				Family/Friends to Contact in Emergency

Use blanks to fill in other essential information pertinent to your family situation.

Endnotes

Chapter 1

1. "What is Caregiving? Utah Caregiving Coalition," www://utahcares.org/?s=provision.
2. June Hunt. *Caregiving: A Privilege: Not a Prison*. Dallas: Hope for the Heart, 2015.
3. *When God Sends Help, Don't Ask Questions.* Senior News. 13 Jan 2017.
4. "Home Safety Checklist." *Consumer Product Safety Commission Safety for Older Consumers,* www.cpsc.gov/PageFiles/122038/701.pdf.

Chapter 2

1. Tara Siegel Bernard. "The Talk You Didn't Have with Your Parents Could Cost." *New York Times*, 24 May 2013, www.nytimes.com/2013/05/25/your-money/aging-parents-and-children-shouldtalk-about-finances.html.
2. "Understanding the Differences Between a Will and a Trust," *Elder Law Net*, www.elderlawanswers.com/understanding-the-differences-between-a-will-and-a-trust-7888.
3. "Advance CARE Planning." National Institute on Aging, www.nia.nih.gov/health/advance-care-planning-healthcare-directives.
4. Medical Definition of HIPAA. www.medicinenet, www.medicinenet.com/script/main/art.asp?articlekey=31785.
5. Kathleen Michon. "First Steps to Managing an Elder's Finances." *NOLO*, www.nolo.com/legal-encyclopedia/helping-seniors-manage-money-finances-32268.html.
6. "Caring for Your Parents: Caregiver's Handbook." *PBS*, www.pbs.org/wgbh/caringforyourparents/handbook.

Chapter 3

1. "Advocate." *Merriam-Webster*," www.merriamwebster.com/dictionary/advocate.
2. "Alzheimer's Disease." National Memory Screening Program. *Alzheimer's Foundation of America*, www.nationalmemoryscreening.org/alzheimers-definition.php.
3. "What are the Signs of Alzheimer's Disease." *National Institute on Aging U.S. Department of Health and Human Services*, www.nia.nih.gov/health/what-are-signs-alzheimers-disease.
4. Owen Darnell. "Do Not Ask Me to Remember." *The Senior List*, 4 Dec 2015, www.theseniorlist.com/2015/12/do-not-ask-me-to-remember-an-alzheimers-poem.
5. "What Medicare covers." *The Official U.S. Government Site for Medicare*, www.medicare.gov/what-medicare-covers/index.html.

Chapter 4

1. Barbara Brotman. "Older Parents Divulge What It's Like to Leave Home to Live Near Adult Kids." *Chicago Tribune*, 5 June 2015. www.chicagotribune.com/news/ct-elderly-moves-brotman-talk-0608-20150605-story.html.
2. "Paying for Senior Care," www.payingforseniorcare.com.
3. *Assisted Living Today*, www.assistedlivingtoday.com.
4. Larry Beresford and Elisabeth Kubler-Ross. *Hospice Handbook: A Complete Guide.* Canada Limited: Little, Brown and Company, 1993.
5. Susan Barton. "Knowing the Difference Between Hospice and Palliative Care." *The Billings Gazette*, 25 June 2013, billingsgazette.com/lifestyles/health-med-fit/knowing-the-difference-between-hospice-and-palliative-care/article_08a95f08-ea1d-54c3-a970-ee86474ad470.html.

Chapter 5

1. Stanton Berg. "Negative Noise and Alzheimer's." *June K. Berg: A Journey Through Alzheimer's.* 28 May 2008, www.junebergalzheimers.com/care-practices/negative-Noise.
2. Greene, Patti. *Answer Me: Developing a Heart for Prayer.* Bloomington: Westbow, 2016.

3. Four Spiritual Laws English. *CRU*, www.crustore.org/fourlawseng.htm. 5 Feb 2018.

4. "Begin Your Journey to Peace," www.peacewithgod.net.

Chapter 6

1. "What to Expect When Your Loved One is Dying." WebMD, www.webmd.com.

2. Clark Randall. "Things to Do Immediately After a Loved One Dies." *USA Today*, 24 Oct 2015. www.usatoday.com/story/money/personalfinance/2015/10/24/credit-dotcom-after-loved-one-dies-finances/74263212.

3. "Advance CARE Planning." National Institute on Aging. www.nia.nih.gov/health/advance-care-planning-healthcare-directives.

Bibliography

"Advocate." *Merriam-Webster*," www.merriam-webster.com/dictionary/advocate. Accessed 8 May 2017.

"Alzheimer's Disease." National Memory Screening Program. *Alzheimer's Foundation of America*, www.nationalmemoryscreening.org/alzheimers-definition.php. Accessed 5 Feb 2018.

Assisted Living Today, www.assistedlivingtoday.com. Accessed 5 May 2017.

Barton, Susan. "Knowing the Difference Between Hospice and Palliative Care." *The Billings Gazette*, 25 June 2013, billingsgazette.com/lifestyles/health-med-fit/knowing-the-difference-between-hospice-and-palliative-care/article_08a95f08-eald-54c3-a970-ee86474ad470.html. Accessed 13 Feb. 2018.

"Begin Your Journey to Peace," www.peacewithgod.net. Accessed 10 May 2017.

Beresford, Larry and Elisabeth Kubler-Ross. *Hospice Handbook: A Complete Guide.* Canada Limited: Little, Brown and Company, 1993.

Berg, Stanton. "Negative Noise and Alzheimer's." *June K. Berg: A Journey Through Alzheimer's.* 28 May 2008, www.junebergalzheimers.com/care-practices/

Negative-Noise. Accessed 13 Feb 2018.

Bernard, Tara Siegel. "The Talk You Didn't Have with Your Parents Could Cost." *New York Times*, 24 May 2013, www.nytimes.com/2013/05/25/your-money/aging-parents-and-children-shouldtalk-about-finances.html. Accessed 22 April 2017.

Birkbeck, Rob. "Traditional church and tower in China." *Found*, Lightstock, 1 Feb 2018. www.lightstock.com.

Brotman, Barbara. "Older Parents Divulge What It's Like to Leave Home to Live Near Adult Kids." *Chicago Tribune*, 5 June 2015. www.chicagotribune.com/news/ct-elderly-moves-brotman-talk-0608-20150605-story.html. Accessed 22 April 2017.

"Caring for Your Parents: The Caregiver's Handbook." *PBS*,
www.pbs.org/wgbh/caringforyourparents/handbook. Accessed 19 Apr
2017.

Darnell, Owen. "Do Not Ask Me to Remember." *The Senior List*, 4 Dec 2015,
www.theseniorlist.com/2015/12/do-not-ask-me-to-remember-an-poem.
Accessed Feb 5 2018.

Four Spiritual Laws English. *CRU*, www.crustore.org/fourlawseng.htm. 5 Feb
2018.

Greene, Patti. *Answer Me: Developing a Heart for Prayer*. Bloomington:
WestBow, 2016.

Hebrew-Greek Key Word Study Bible. Ed. Spiros Zodhiates. Chattanooga: AMG,
2008.

"Home Safety Checklist." *Consumer Product Safety Commission Safety for Older
Consumers*, www.cpsc.gov/PageFiles/122038/701.pdf. Accessed 19 Apr
2017.

Hunt, June. *Caregiving: A Privilege: Not a Prison*. Dallas: Hope for the Heart,
2015.

McGovern, Sue. *What Everyone Should Know About Hospice*. St. Meinrad:
Abbey Press. 2004.

Medical Definition of HIPAA. www.medicinenet,
www.medicinenet.com/script/main/art.asp?articlekey=31785. Accessed
8 Feb 2018.

Michon, Kathleen. "First Steps to Managing an Elder's Finances." *NOLO*,
www.nolo.com/legal-encyclopedia/helping-seniors-manage-money-
finances-32268.html. Accessed 22 April 2017.

"Paying for Senior Care," www.payingforseniorcare.com. Accessed 5 May
2017.

Petersen, Brian A. "Vintage power outlets in a barn in South Dakota." *Found*, 1
Feb 2018, Lightstock, www.lightstock.com.

"Preparing for the Death of a Loved One." *National Caregiver's Library*,
www.caregiverslibrary.org. Accessed 15 Oct 2016.

Randall, Clark. "Things to Do Immediately After a Loved One Dies." *USA Today*, 24 Oct 2015. www.usatoday.com/story/money/personalfinance/2015/10/24/credit-dotcom-after-loved-one-dies-finances/74263212. Accessed 15 Oct 2016.

Real Findo. "A man's hand punches in numbers on a calculator sitting atop of bills." *Found,* 1 Feb 2018, Lightstock, www.lightstock.com.

Redman Creative. "An elderly couple driving a red convertible on a curvy road." *Found,* 14 Feb 2018, Lightstock, www.lightstock.com.

Ruch, Jennifer. "Elderly woman looking at her pill box." *Found,* 1 Feb 2018, Lightstock, www.lightstock.com.

Totra, Dallas. "Grandmother and granddaughter." *Found,* 14 Feb 2018, Lightstock, www.lightstock.com.

"Understanding the Differences Between a Will and a Trust." *Elder Law Net,* www.elderlawanswers.com/understanding-the-differences-between-a-will-and-a-trust-7888. Accessed 8 Feb 2018.

Wang, Neely. "Flowers growing under a cross glowing in sunlight." *Found,* Lightstock, 1 Feb 2018, www.lightstock.com.

"What are the Signs of Alzheimer's Disease." *National Institute on Aging U.S. Department of Health and Human Services,* www.nia.nih.gov/health/what-are-signs-alzheimers-disease. Accessed 22 Apr. 2017.

"What is Caregiving? Utah Caregiving Coalition," www://utahcares.org/?s=provision. Accessed 19 Apr 2017.

"What Medicare covers." *The Official U.S. Government Site for Medicare,* www.medicare.gov/what-medicare-covers/index.html. Accessed 13 Feb 2018.

"What to Expect When Your Loved One is Dying." WebMD, www.webmd.com. Accessed 15 Oct 2016.

When God Sends Help, Don't Ask Questions. Senior News. 13 Jan 2017.

Young, Lisa F. "Caring nursing home orderly pops a wheelie with an elderly man's wheelchair." *Found,* 2017, Shutterstock. www.shutterstock.com.

Notes

Notes

Notes